OFF THE MEDS

The Surprising Path to Ending Suffering from Asthma and Allergies

By Michelle Brown, JD AP

Copyright

Nothing in this book is suggested to have you avoid seeing a board-certified physician for a proper diagnosis for your health concerns. These statements have not been evaluated by the FDA and are intended for educational purposes only. All recommendations for essential oils are based on third-party research for essential oils and their effectiveness when used for the above ailments. See PubMed for references to some of those studies. Take personal responsibility based on complete information for your healthcare.

Dr. Brown only recommends CPTG essential oils from Doterra as they are the only essential on the market that show superior quality, growing and harvesting techniques as well as being grown in indigenous regions of the world. Further, the Doterra essential oils contain no synthetic chemicals or preservatives and are tested extensively. There are many essential oils in the marketplace today but not many companies that have set such high standards and produce therapeutic benefit. Always check your essential oil bottles for supplement facts and if you don't have an oil that can be used for internal use don't use it.

Author's photo courtesy of Ashley Tiseo, Aurora Jade Photography

Advance Praise

This kind of effort put forth by Dr. Michelle is extraordinary as the learning journey is very difficult for Chinese people to let alone for her being an American to accomplish the whole journey. She even gave up practicing the law but practices TCM instead. I believe TCM is becoming an inseparable part of her life.
Dr. Peng Lei, Director of Traditional Chinese Medicine, Kowloon Hospital, Suzhou China

Dr. Michelle's accomplishments remind me of a Chinese Saying "墙内开花墙外香 qiang nei kai hua qiang wai xiang" literally translated "Blooming inside but perfuming outside", meaning some accomplishments are easily known outside its own unit. In Michelle's story, the way she appreciates and benefits from TCM is way more than most Chinese people. I hope Americans can benefit from this book
Dr. Zeng Cong Jun, Vice Chief Radiologist, Kowloon Hospital, Suzhou China

"This book is so important because it is a significant look at the current American medical system, and it comes at the right time. It works as a guide for all patients, giving its purpose remarkable value. "
Dr. He Chong, MD (China) AP Fort Lauderdale, FL

Dedication

When I first met my husband, I could not believe I met someone so kind, caring, and awesome. I knew he was an angel sent to me from GOD. Everything that has happened in my life since I met him is because of him. I would have never of had the opportunity to change my life without him and for that, I am eternally grateful. I will love you forever!

Table of Contents

Chinese Proverb

If you are planning for a year sow rice.

If you are planning for a decade plant some trees.

If you are planning for a lifetime educate people.

Unknown Author

Keep educating people. One person at a time can make a difference.

Chapter 1

The Problem

I was the first person to get an advanced degree in my family. I had the perfect husband, a great job as an attorney, and two awesome dachshunds! At 42 years old, my career was taking off and I was earning excellent money and getting interesting cases. It was a lot of work and stressful too, but I loved it. Butch, my husband had a great job, making good money, full benefits, running an automotive factory. Almost everyone in our family lived close to each other in a small town in Indiana. In fact, no one in his family has ever left Indiana before. Everything was going great! Butch and I talked often about how to retire as early as possible and began to purchase rental properties for extra income in addition to the full-time jobs we had. We both worked on cleaning them, painting them and getting them to a point where we could rent them or resell them. In 2003 after sanding the floors of a 100-year-old property, I began to have respiratory problems. I soon was diagnosed with asthma and allergies. I was told the problems were never to be cured, and to take Advair, Singulair, Zyrtec, Benadryl, Prednisone, use a rescue inhaler as needed and take

Protonix for acid reflux that you may or may not have, and have Pulmicort on standby if you need an at home breathing treatment! The doctor said I would need all these drugs or the rest of my life. I was warned if you stop these drugs your lungs could fail, and you could die. I remember calling my cousin who has had asthma from childhood and she confirmed that this was her treatment too. I could not accept this. From the beginning of the diagnosis and treatments I felt worse, and the answer every time I went to the pulmonologist was," let's try a different drug, let's do allergy injections, you always have your prednisone, try more Benadryl". Never was there an alternative or complementary option offered. I didn't know what to do. One day for the first time ever, I read the patient package inserts to the drugs I had been taking and I had many of the side effects listed on the PPI. There never was an end to the drugs, in fact, I always left my Dr.'s office with a bag of drug samples. I can't believe now that I never looked at what I was told to take, I just trusted my Doctor and western medicine. I began to worry what the long-term use of prednisone would do to my body, and what the other reported side effects from the other drugs were doing. My cousin is 8 years younger than me and already has osteoporosis, her

11

doctor told her most likely from years of prednisone use. I was scared and wanted to fight this disease and the drugs but didn't know how. I also participated in a study at the National Jewish hospital for a few months. I thought this would help but I soon found out they were willing to give information about asthma and drugs but when I asked about how to get off these drugs the answer was that's it is not possible. It was apparent to me they were working for the drug company that makes Advair. Chronic sinus infections, chest colds, sore throat, itchy nose, coughing and hoarse voice with dark circles under my eyes were a common occurrence for almost two years. I was sick or didn't feel great most of the time. I was struggling and not getting better. The cost of the drugs was astronomical too. I keep asking myself, what can I do to get off these drugs and cure myself? Then in June of 2005, Butch got a job offer that would change everything. He was promoted to General Manager of an Elastomer and Rubber Manufacturing Company in Mainland China! We were moving to a third world country! Shortly after deciding to move to China my friend Christine told me that I should try acupuncture and Chinese medicine when I get to China and that her sister as an acupuncture physician in Seattle. This was the first time I had ever heard of acupuncture or anyone having a career in this type of medicine. Moving to China was never on my radar either! I was about to begin a new journey! I think I have found a way to finally get off these drugs and get well. I want you to know that I am not opposed to western allopathic medicine, I am opposed to overprescribing of drugs and doctors that don't combine complementary medicine into their practice. You need to know when to question your doctor about appropriate treatments and not be afraid to make your own informed healthcare decision. I hope you will find a solution for your asthma and allergies in this book and will be part of the solution for the future of medicine. Chinese Lotus flowers grow in the muck and emerge as a beautiful flower! You too can pull yourself from the muck and emerge as a beautiful healthy flower.

Chapter 2

My Story September 2018

It has been 13 years since my life changed forever. Waiting for Cindy, my Chinese daughter, to get off the plane at Regional Southwest airport brought back so many memories of my life in China! I have had so many requests to share my story and this has finally led me to write it all down. I hope if you ever have an opportunity to do something so different from what you know, that scares you, that excites you, you take advantage of it, it will open your mind to new thinking and adventures that will change you for the better for the rest of your life.

June 2005 Exploration

June 2005 was a crazy month with Butch announcing that his company was going to build some factories in Mainland China and he was interested in heading up the project. I was blown away because I never had China on my radar. Where was China? We had a lot of questions. We were so excited and scared about the possibilities and adventure. We were really unsure about what to do! Then within 2 weeks, Butch was leaving for a 2-week trip to China. He arrived in Shanghai with two coworkers and began an intensive exploration trip to

Suzhou, Ningbo, and Dalian looking for a place to build a new state of the art manufacturing and rubber mixing facility. We got our first experience of being in two different locations with 12 hours' time difference. We only had a very short window every day to talk. When I was working, he was sleeping, when he was working, I was sleeping. Back then we didn't have iPhones or good internet. Communication was a challenge. Butch's first impression of China was that there were many new building projects and some roads were built. There were so many bicycles. He was really surprised! He saw so many building cranes, he named them "The new bird of China"! We still say that every time we see a building crane anywhere we go! When he got back, he was so excited about the possibility of doing something so big, so far away from our reality, and something so different. He gave the company a presentation about the project and then we waited! In August, we were asked to go to China to look for a place to live and decide if we could live there. We planned a 10-day trip and left at the end of August. We arrived in Shanghai at the end of August after a 13-hour flight. It was so hot when we arrived, and I was sick again with a respiratory cold. It was pure chaos at the airport, more people than you can imagine! As we walked through immigration and exited the arrival gate there were thousands of people waiting to greet family friends and business associates. Everyone there had black hair and 5 feet tall. At 5'5" tall I was taller than most of the men there! We were told all Americans look alike. We laughed a lot about that because we thought all Chinese people looked the same when we first got to China too. In addition, we were told we are too fat! There were very few Caucasian faces there. We didn't speak Chinese then, and there was so much noise, it was so confusing. The language barrier was difficult, and we knew right away we had to learn to speak Chinese. As we walked through the door, we were greeted by the company driver, Mr. Chen, who drove us to Suzhou for our first meeting with the government officials. He was holding a card with our name on it. Butch knew him right away as he had met him in June during his first trip. Mr. Chen was my first experience with a mainland Chinese person. He had worked for the Company for a few years, but only had his driver's license for a short period of time. Not many cars were owned by private people and not many people could even drive. The main mode of transport was the bus, bicycle or an electric bike. It was unbelievable that we had been driving 30 plus years and we were being driven by someone who just got their driver's license. Mr. Chen wore white gloves to drive the car. He had never been to Suzhou before as it was a 2.5-hour drive from Shanghai. This was very typical of most Chinese people at the time. They stayed in their home towns. The highway was a two-lane road in good condition. We made good time until we got off on the Suzhou exit and Mr. Chen was lost. After a few phone calls, we finally found our way to the hotel and after 24 hours of traveling, we got to our hotel. We found out right away everyone has a cell phone in China and very few people have a land line. We arrived in the evening and I was surprised that the city and the buildings were lit up like Christmas trees. We stayed at the only foreign hotel at the time in Suzhou, the Ramada Inn. When we arrived, we found out very quickly that no one really spoke English. They could speak a few words but communication at a deep level wasn't going to happen. Our room was clean and adequate, but the bed was hard as a rock. It was like a board with a blanket sewn on it. There was no pillow top mattress here. The next day we were picked up at the hotel by the Suzhou New District government officials. We were told that Suzhou was a small tier two city, with 8 million people. At the time, we were living in a rural town in

Indiana with only 15,000 people. I had never met a communist before and all of sudden I was in a room with 5 of them. They asked us a lot of questions about our jobs and what we were like. They were being very guarded when we asked questions and we never felt like we got the full answer or even an answer. We were taken to a few different apartments and condos in the new district and found one that we thought could work. We went to lunch then dinner and didn't get much time alone on this trip. At the end of dinner, I was told I had a teaching job at the law school when I arrived in Suzhou for my 4-year stay. I was shocked, but I was told that I had more experience in law than anyone in the whole country of China, as the practice of law was a newly authorized profession, and that they could learn from me. They asked me to teach American business law and to prepare a plan to teach it. I said OK. Eating was a huge challenge and we soon found out that Chinese food in China was not the same as in the USA. Everything had bones and heads of animals in it and fat was not trimmed from the meat. It was going to be interesting for sure. The smells of the foods were so strong and putrid and the tastes so different, I wasn't sure I was going to find things I liked to eat. This soon changed though. We did some sightseeing at the pagoda at the hotel, then we had to leave for Shanghai to visit the corporate office. We really didn't get a good feeling of what living in Suzhou would be like. This trip went by so fast that the next thing we knew we were back in Angola, IN. We were so excited about the possibility of this adventure. To do something new, so far away from our reality and that was so different was the biggest thing we have ever done. At this point, though we were not sure the project was a go and we didn't have a signed contract with the company. There were a lot of things to consider. I had a law practice with employees, all of our family and friends lived fairly close to us and we had never lived in a foreign country. I was really concerned because the air pollution which was really bad there and wondered how I would survive with my respiratory challenges. Now, all we could do was wait and see what happens. The next 3.5 months were very stressful with the sale of our house, the sale of my law practice and my grandfather dying just 3 weeks before we moved to China. It went by so fast and on December 17th we left Angola to spend two weeks in our Florida home before leaving for China on 12/26/05. I would spend 3 weeks in China and then return to transition my law practice to the new owner, and then permanently move in

July 2006. This is my story, I hope you enjoy it. My husband has been a huge catalyst in my life, making it so awesome and exciting, giving me the courage to change everything I knew to find a better life.

December 2005

We arrived in Florida at ten in the morning on the 17th of December, how nice it was to leave 22 degrees and find 75 degrees and sunshine. It has only been 14 days since my grandfather died and I was having second thoughts about moving to China. I had always told my grandmother I wanted her to live with me if anything ever happened to Pappy. I always had a feeling that he would go first but I had spent the weekend with him just 2 weeks before he passed, and I just didn't think he was dying. As I look back at the last picture I have of him, I can see he had sadness in his eyes. I was so sad he died. I spent so much time as a kid at their home and wanted to live with them full-time. I know they both loved me very much. And I loved them. My parents picked us up at the airport in Florida and Nanny came to stay with me for a few days before I left for China. We had a great time cooking pierogis, knitting scarves and having her crochet bear-shaped cleaning scrubs. I asked her so many times about coming to live with me, but she would not have it. She wanted to go back to Pennsylvania every day. She ended up spending the winter in Florida and then going back to her home by herself. Two weeks flew by and on December 26, 2005, we left for China! We had talked to Vivian, the Company assistant to Butch, 2 days prior and our furniture had arrived at our condo in Suzhou. Vivian and another employee had unpacked our boxes and got our place all organized. The flight over was very stressful as it was running late, and the airline's employees were very uptight trying to load people very fast. We decided to take our nephew Adam to China for a two-week visit. When we got to our seats, we found out that Adam's seat was given to someone else. After a bit of confusion, Adam got to sit in business class and Butch and I sat together in economy plus. I set my watch ahead and 14 hours later we arrived in Shanghai, China. Just like the first time we went there Mr. Chen was smiling and waving as we walked thru the doors. He had been patiently waiting to pick us up and drive us to Suzhou. We had only slept a little and arrived at 4:56 pm, exhausted. Now we had a 2-hour drive to our new home. After Mr. Chen got lost two times, we finally made it there. It was so cold when we arrived, but the girls had organized our house, so we could get right in bed and get some sleep. At 11:00 pm after losing one whole day we were here! We didn't read, write or speak Chinese and had no idea what was ahead of us. We were up at 6:00 am after only 7 hours of sleep, but we had a lot of excitement and adrenaline flowing and felt pretty good. Today we had planned to go to the grocery store and try to find some items for our new house. The condo was a 3-story building connected to another building to the right. It was heated by a small wall unit on each floor and the units were not big enough to keep the place warm. The first floor was so cold you had to wear a winter coat and you could see your breath when you talked. It also had a weird sewer smell that we found out was very common in China. We had arrived in Suzhou. It was so cold and damp. Our townhouse was new construction with wood and marble floors. It had three levels and a spiral staircase. Our assistant, Vivian, was her English name. Vivian was a young girl with a strong cold personality. The reality of what we just did was apparent immediately when we realized we did not read, write or speak Chinese and we had to rely on this stranger. Our first issue happened the next day. The house alarm went off and we could not shut it off. This was because we could not read Chinese. We called Vivian who came right over and shut off the alarm. A short time later that day we could not figure out how to use the dishwasher or washing machine. When I decided to take a shower the water was ice cold because Butch had dumped our solar water heater by mistake. I started to cry uncontrollably. It was three days of complete emotional breakdown. Vivian did not know what to do with me. She kept saying "you cry like a baby". She was unable to understand how far we had come and what we had given up coming to a place where we could not communicate. I had never felt so scared and helpless before. After three days I realized I had to survive, so we started finding resources to help us adjust. The first thing we did was take a trip to the appliance store to find templates in English for the appliances. This helped us so much. The second thing was to ban Butch from touching the solar heater! My nephew who had just graduated from photography school came with us for that first month we were in China. He was so excited to go out and take pictures. It was a huge surprise when he came back from his first outing-- he had photographed a man pulling his pants down by a bridge and defecating in plain view! I could not believe what I was seeing. It wasn't long after that we experienced people urinating and spitting in the streets

23

everywhere. It became a daily annoyance to be in an elevator and have someone spit down by my feet or be walking and someone would squat down by a tree and pee. My first respiratory problem happened the second day we were in China when we got into our company car and the driver had a cologne bottle on the dashboard. I started coughing and sneezing. I could not stand to smell any perfume, cigarette smoke or anything that had a fragrance. Smoking was everywhere. The next day I was able to get a recommendation from the Human Resources Manager at the company about a famous local acupuncture physician in Suzhou. She immediately took me there. You didn't need an appointment. It was first come first serve for treatment. I met Dr. Ouyang Basi that cold day in December for my first treatment. I didn't know then that he would become one of my teachers and I would work with him in that same clinic where I got my treatment. I remember telling my husband that I'm an attorney that helps people solve problems every day, so I should be able to figure out how to cure myself. After my first acupuncture treatment, I knew I could get well and made a decision to follow Dr. Ouyang's advice, to get off all the western drugs and tonify and strengthen my lung function. I didn't even know what that meant. I was scared, but I told myself I have all the medicine I brought from the USA if I need them. I was still coming out of the allopathic medicine brainwashing in which I was raised. I received six treatments in my first month in China and was beginning to feel better. I had stopped my medicines but felt a lot of tightness and constriction in my lungs. I had been on these medicines for almost 2 years, and I wasn't going back. The day was so liberating when I quit these drugs but I was a little worried because this isn't how I was educated about medicine. Most people in the USA have a similar experience unless your parents had been hippies and were against the establishment. A month went by quickly and I was just getting used to the time zone change (12 hours ahead of USA) when I had to go back to Indiana to finish the transition of the sale of my law practice to the new owner. Butch remained in China and began his job to set up a factory from ground zero. The time went by fast and in July 2006 I arrived back in Suzhou for the almost four-year adventure that completely changed my life forever. Before returning to China, I found a medical Doctor who had left the mainstream drug pushing practice and had just opened an acupuncture clinic in Fort Wayne, Indiana, about 40 miles from my house. Her hope was to make a difference in healthcare. I began seeing her weekly for acupuncture treatments and was making good progress until I decided to get a flu shot, tetanus and hepatitis vaccine. This was one of the worst decisions I had ever made. I didn't know at the time that vaccines contain a lot of preservatives, mercury, and other fillers that can cause bad outcomes to people who take them. I began to wheeze, had a rash all over my body and had lesions forming on my arms and legs. I was so itchy and uncomfortable. I hadn't realized at the time that this was a dangerous situation. It wasn't until I went to my doctor's office to get some papers signed for my living permit in China that a nurse at the office realized that I was in respiratory distress. That day I had to get a shot of prednisone again. I was so disturbed. I vowed then to find a way to get well and never take these vaccines or drugs again. I will never get another vaccine. I am not opposed to western medicine, I am opposed to the drug pushing practices that don't identify and treat the underlying cause of disease.

Cindy

I met Cindy for the first time in April 2006 when I took a quick 10-day trip to Singapore and China for our seventh wedding anniversary. Butch had arranged for me to meet this young Chinese girl who was hired to be my assistant and translator. I will never forget the day I first saw her. She came to my house in the morning to meet me. From the second I opened the door and saw this tiny black-haired, black-eyed girl looking at me with a huge smile I knew it would be okay in China. Cindy was an English major and was so happy to meet me. I found out later that although Cindy had studied English for many years, I was the first American she had ever seen. Cindy was graduating from college in June and would be looking for her first job. I fell in love with Cindy immediately and felt like she could have been my child. I cannot explain the feeling that came over me, but I called Cindy my daughter from that day forward. She agreed immediately to be my assistant. We began speaking and shopping and learning together. When I returned to China permanently in July Cindy began working with me three days a week. In August, we made some big changes. The month of July was my second full month in China and I started to experience what it was like living in a foreign country. Having blond curly hair, blue eyes and white skin, I stood out like a sore thumb. All of our neighbors were Chinese. Many of the older Chinese women would come to our front door and try and get a glimpse of me. One day when Cindy was coming in, she was approached by a woman that wanted to know how old I was because she saw my husband and thought he was too old for me. Cindy assured her that there was not that much difference in our ages and it was okay. Another time I found a few neighbors in my garden looking around. The couple next door was impossible. They constantly parked in our driveway, blocking our garage and were always yelling so loud we could hear them through the walls. We tried to make friends with them by giving them some oranges, but I found out later I gave them four oranges which is an unlucky number and it scared them. While this was happening, Cindy had been kicked out of her new apartment one night by a dishonest landlord who would not fix the leaking plumbing and faulty air conditioner. She was so scared because she lived two hours from her parents and did not know what to do. I immediately got her to the safety of our townhouse and we began working on a plan that would help us all out. The prior week I had gone to a yoga presentation that was given by my new yoga teacher in the countryside. While I was at yoga, I met a German family that told me about the only single-family homes that were built in the Suzhou New

District (SND). It sounded amazing. I decided to go look at them the next day. I asked my driver, Zhu, to take me there. Tian Ling Feng Jing was the name of the complex. It was a gated community at the base of Ling Yen Mountain. There were 100 houses built in an old fruit tree farm. It was beautiful, and I loved it immediately. We found out there were three new homes available for rent. I immediately called Butch and we discussed the situation and decided to try to negotiate a new rental lease. We also asked Cindy to move in with us. It was a win/win situation. We could have a native speaker help us with our language barrier and we could help her live in a safe place. I immediately called her and asked her to consider it. The next day I took her to the new house and she could not believe her luck. We negotiated a 3-year rental with her help and within a week we all moved to a four-bedroom, four-bath house with a garage and a pool. It was 5000 square feet. The house was perfectly designed to give us all privacy in a beautiful location.

The Beginning Months

July, August, and September and October 2006

July

I immediately began my treatments at the Traditional Medicine Hospital once I was permanently relocated to Suzhou. The hospital was very old, dirty and the treatment rooms were open so anyone walking by could see you getting your treatment. The tables were a board with a very thin pad on top. There were no clean sheets, and everyone laid on the same pad. The needles for Chinese patients in this hospital were reused. I brought my own needles for my treatments. I also had to pay first and then get treatment. Most Americans would not have wanted to get treatment at this hospital. I had no choice at the time and I made the best of it. I was feeling better every day, even though I was living in a place that has extreme air pollution. I really wondered how this could be. At the beginning of my treatments, I was so scared about getting needles. Now I was looking forward to my treatments.

August

In August, I started my new job at Suzhou University Law School teaching American Business Law. On my first day of class over 100 students came to my class, I think just to see me. The first student to introduce herself to me was a representative of the Communist party. She wanted me to know she was there. After the first class, I had only 20 students who were the best English speakers. I found out quickly that law students in China are not as articulate as Americans and are very reserved. They wanted me to write everything down on the chalkboard, so they could copy it. Asking them to learn by the Socratic Method wasn't going to fly. It turned out to be a good experience, but I didn't want to return the following semester because I felt that there was no interest in the faculty doing projects together. The whole time I was there I never made friends with any Chinese teachers, only an American man from California who was teaching there like me. The dean took us out to lunch once, but I didn't get the feeling he was really interested in what I was doing.

September

In September, I attended my first ex-pat meeting where I met people from all over the world who were living in Suzhou. There were two American women and one Chinese American with whom I became friends. Rae, the Chinese American women, will forever be in my gratitude. She really helped me to understand the culture, gave me reading sources about

Chinese history and took me to the first western and Chinese medicine hospital that had just opened up in the SSIP district (Suzhou Singapore Industrial Project). This was a turning point for me because I met the director of Chinese medicine, Peng Lei, who became a dear friend as well as an inspiration for my change of career, but I didn't know it yet. At that meeting, I also met a German woman who was a medical doctor in Germany. She had a great interest in studying Chinese medicine while living in Suzhou and invited Rae and me to study Chinese medicine and acupuncture at the first-ever training program for foreigners. At the time, I was interested but didn't have any medical experience. She assured us that it would be ok and that we would start from ground zero and learn everything. Rae agreed to be the translator for the class and the following April we started class with approximately 20 women from 20 different countries. I wanted to satisfy my curiosity about how this Chinese medicine and acupuncture was able to help me get better. I had only known a system where you go to the doctor, take drugs, sometimes for life and that's it. With Chinese medicine, you are given an acupuncture treatment protocol and herbs based on what your tongue looks like and your pulse feels like. I have to be honest, I really didn't understand anything I was being told, partly due to the language barrier but also because the lingo was so different from what Americans learn about western medicine. I really thought that I was studying Chinese medicine as a hobby and would not leave the practice of law. I was just having faith that it would help me because I would not go back to the drugs. This brainwashing was always in the back of my mind in the beginning. I started seeing Peng Lei and her doctors at Kowloon Hospital in the SSIP that September and was experiencing really great results. This hospital was a western medical center with the most advanced diagnostic tools and cancer treatment facilities. The Chinese medicine department was a small part of the hospital, but they used new needles on everyone and the rooms were separated by a curtain. If you wanted clean sheets though, you had to bring your own. I began adding treatments for my foot and back pain and started meeting doctors from the hospital. It was a magical time to start experiencing so many different things. I started teaching English at my husband's company and to the doctors at Kowloon hospital and we began getting invitations from Chinese people to go out to dinner and visit historical sites. Dr. Colin Zeng, one of my first English students, has become a great friend and has taught me so much about imaging. I was starting to adjust. It really took until the end of 2006 to acclimate to this environment. It was so different from what we had known. The food was so different, we experienced a lot of digestion problems and we could not get many western things like paper towels, pasta, and butter in the beginning. This changed in 2007 when a German grocery store opened in our area, alleviating the need to drive 2.5 hrs. to Shanghai for groceries.

October

In October 2006, we went to Cindy's hometown of Changzhou for the October holiday. She showed us around and we created quite a stir at a local Buddhist monastery. People were trying to touch us and take our pictures. Most of the people there had never seen or met a foreign person before. I was amazed at how nice people were considering the communist rhetoric that we were "Foreign Devils". It was here that a Buddhist Monk approached Cindy and asked her if he could read my "Bazi". The Bazi looks at a person's 4 pillars of destiny. I agreed, and this is when I was told I carry the star of medicine in my destiny and I will switch careers. I really didn't give it much thought as I had planned to practice law when I went back to the USA. Studying medicine in China was just something to do for fun. In fact, I had just been approached by a Danish consulting firm that was looking for someone with my legal experience to help them with a few legal projects concerning business law.

What was it like to live in China?

I have been asked many times "what was it like to live in China"? My first response is to say it was so life changing on so many levels. It was different, dirty, uncivilized at times, crowded, impressive, there is so much history, parts of the country are beautiful, the cities are huge, change can be seen, it's not a free speech country, religion is suppressed, there are a lot of people there, people are very disorderly and at times people are cold to each other. It was an adventure of a lifetime. Finding a cure for my health concerns in and of itself should be my main highlight, but I have to say that experiencing the culture, meeting so many new people, learning a new language, yes I learned to speak Mandarin, getting an opportunity to retire for 6 years at a young age, travelling all over Asia, eating different foods, working in an orphanage, teaching English, learning about medicine, getting my Captain's boating license for China, and so much more, they have been the synergistic link to the experience. I left there having made lifelong friends with people who really were not so different than me, living there made me feel like maybe I'd been there before, and I was just like them now.

Chapter 3

Solutions to Make the Change for your Healthcare

If you are suffering from asthma, allergies, or other health concerns and don't know what to do to improve your health, you have come to the right place. In this chapter, we will discuss the steps to take to begin to heal your body. You don't have to go to China as I did. My last visit to a pulmonologist was in March of 2006. After I had my exam the doctor told me my lung function was normal and to keep doing what I was doing. I told him that is great news because I hadn't taken any of the drugs he prescribed for approximately 3 months and I had been getting acupuncture and herbal medicine and felt cured. He told me he didn't understand how complementary medicine worked but felt there was: "something to it". He said "I really can't believe I misdiagnosed you", maybe your blood was attacking itself" and asked if he could run a blood sample and check it. I agreed and about 20 minutes later his theory went up in smoke when he checked my blood. The results were fine. To this day I don't understand what he was looking for, but I never went back, and I have never had an asthma attack since. I have had colds but never needed any of those drugs again. I can tolerate going out in public and don't feel hypersensitive to smells. I don't experience any symptoms when the season changes and have not had any allergy attacks like I used to have. Respiratory diseases like asthma and allergies are really misunderstood in allopathic western medicine. If you are like me, you have been going to see a pulmonologist for a while with no major improvements or you are now beginning to have side effects from the medications you are taking. Don't worry, there are solutions. Stop taking the flu shot and vaccines. These vaccines contain chemicals and other ingredients that cause cancer. The cancer-causing chemicals are mostly heavy metals that disrupt the nervous system, endocrine system, digestive system, and epithelial tissue. The vaccines cause the body to produce antibodies to the disease but are not strong enough to stop people from getting the disease or stopping it for a lifetime. The vaccines also contain DNA and RNA from animals, formaldehyde, anti-freeze-like compounds and fetal tissue. Work on making your own immunity thru healthy living. Don't be guided by the fear that is taught to doctors. Remember we all die from something it's how we live prior to that time that matters. Be informed.

Things to DO:

First- Find a board-certified Physician that practices Acupuncture and Chinese medicine. NCCAOM is the National Certification Commission for Acupuncture and Oriental Medicine. You can search the database to find physicians in your area and research their areas of specialties to find the right fit for you. Be sure to find a physician that is board certified as the requirements for physicians has changed a lot over the years and there are many acupuncturists that have not studied western medicine or injection therapy and have been grandfathered into the system. These people are acupuncturists and may not be able to order specialized testing, lab work, homeopathic medicines or vitamin therapy due to lack of training. They focus on needling the body which could help, but most likely will not be able to treat the whole picture of a person's deficiency. There are also many chiropractors and medical doctors that take a training course to be able to do acupuncture, but they provide a totally different service than Acupuncture Physicians practicing Chinese medicine do.

Second- Schedule an appointment and get an examination. For your initial appointment bring complete medical history and any reports you have from your medical doctor. In my clinic, I combine a complete physical exam that is very similar to what you have experienced in a medical doctor's office. The exam consists of 10 different areas of body function, ears, eyes, and nose exam. I will look at the records you brought from your prior doctor's tests. From this information, a diagnosis is made, and a treatment plan is prepared for the patient.

Third- Begin your treatment. Most patients will need at least 10 treatments of acupuncture along with other modalities depending on the health concern that has been presented. Along with the acupuncture, herbal medicines, homeopathic medicines, vitamins, and essential oils are often prescribed. After the initial 10 treatments, an evaluation of your progress is made, and further treatments may be discussed. The length of treatment is usually related to the severity of your condition and the length of time the symptoms have existed.

Fourth- You must have a reasonable expectation for recovery. No form of therapy cures every ailment and Chinese medicine is no different. Additionally, lab tests, imaging, and diagnostic testing may be ordered to help uncover the root cause of your symptoms. The body has an innate ability to heal itself if given the correct tools. Most of my patients are what I call "last resort patients" because I am their last resort. They are all complicated, are taking too many pharmaceuticals, and have been ill for a long time. They have been told they can only take the drugs for their treatment or the doctor does not know what else to do with them. Many of my patients have been told to see psychiatrists because they have complaints that are not understood by western medicine. Some patients tell me that they have asked their doctor about nutrition and they are told by the doctor they know nothing about nutrition and the doctor isn't even interested in trying to learn something that could help their patients. If you have a doctor like this, you should get a new one ASAP. I find it ridiculous that doctors keep repeating this same old mantra but make no effort to augment their education.

Fifth- Start thinking about your body as a weather map. When it is cold out what do you experience? Does extreme heat, dampness, rain, humidity, sunshine, or darkness have an effect on you? Do you have hot flashes, night sweats or feel cold all the time? Write down your symptoms, experiences, and feelings after being exposed to any or all of these conditions and share them with your doctor. This will help with your diagnosis.

Sixth- Start charting what you eat and drink on a daily basis. Food consumption can have an effect on your overall health in ways you may not expect.

Seventh- Start doing light exercise if you are able. Five minutes a day walking or just 1 minute of stretching and breathing in and out can be a start. Medical qi gong, tai chi or yoga can help.

Here is an exercise to try:

Deep Breathing (for improved posture and increased energy levels)

Lay flat on your back on the floor or in your bed. While inhaling, extend your head and neck by elevating the chin to the ceiling. At the same time point your feet down, away from your head. When you reach full inhalation and extension, hold for a count of three and begin to exhale slowly. While exhaling move your chin down to your chest without raising your head or shoulders from the floor or pillow. As you move your chin, bend your feet upward toward your head (your head should reach full extension at the same time you reach complete exhalation)Perform this exercise for one minute- breathing deeply, but at your normal rate Stop the exercise if you become dizzy or light-headed. Start making notes about how you feel before and after this exercise.

Eighth- Set forth a positive intention every day. Release those things that no longer serve you. You are what you think to a certain extent. If you are focused-on illness and negativity, this is what you will experience. You should expect to start making lifestyle changes. This is not magic, voodoo or a miracle cure. This is a system of medicine that has not changed much over the years and is based on prevention by self-healing and regeneration. If you have been to all the western doctors and you are still experiencing symptoms, something has to change for you to get better. If you think you can fool yourself and keep drinking soda, not eating real food, and keep taking drugs to keep yourself healthy, you will be in shock when your body finally has had enough and you have a major health concern like cancer, a stroke, allergic reactions to the meds, organ failure or some other bad outcome from an unhealthy lifestyle. You need to make a commitment to yourself and your treatment, and I promise you will see changes.

Chapter 4

Sick Care Vs Healthcare

The World Health Organization (WHO) definition of health:

"Health is a state of complete physical, mental and social wellbeing and not merely the absence of disease or infirmity".

This definition is what we should strive for in maintaining health at optimal levels. This is my mantra. Make it yours.

To understand where we are today in the USA healthcare system, we have to review the history of the development of medicine. In 1897 the American Medical Association (AMA) was formed. The goal of the AMA was to "promote the science of medicine and betterment of public health". It has a very large political lobbying budget and has been involved in many very controversial positions over the years, calling into question the goals of the organization. In 1948 after WWII the WHO was established with the goal of improving health all over the world. Lab tests and imaging techniques were being offered, new drugs were being developed, heart surgery and transplants began to happen, the US medical school began to be funded for research, and a huge focus was on backing big Pharma. Many of the naturopathic doctors were run out of the country with the anti-German phobias, schools were closed, chiropractors were suppressed or disgraced by the powers that be and homeopathic medicine was ridiculed. Chinese medicine was not even acknowledged until after the 1970's when President Nixon visited China and spoke publicly about acupuncture. In many places like California, where many Asian people lived, Chinese medicine was practiced in back alley treatment rooms to avoid being detected. Today our healthcare system focuses on prescribing drugs to suppress the symptoms of disease instead of determining the root cause of disease, which is even farther away from the WHO definition of health first promulgated in 1948. If you are sick there are thousands of drugs that can be offered but not many physicians offer advice on ways to maintain health and eradicate the disease. Complementary healthcare physicians are popping up here and there but if they are associated with hospital groups, they do not stray far from the drug prescribing paradigm. In fact, many doctors are afraid to offer complimentary health advice, because they will readily admit they don't have any training in that area or they fear criticism from their peers or even firing from the hospitals for which they work. Some will even tell you that they still only had 3-4 hours of nutrition training in their whole career! Almost weekly you will read an article about a complementary physician disappearing or being killed. This is really frightening to think that in this day and age in the USA, physicians are suppressed for sharing healthcare information. It's time to stand up for our rights to have access to all types of medicine and demand integration of complementary medicine into mainstream medicine. When I started medical school in 2009, I was told reform was coming and complementary medicine was going to be integrated with western allopathic medicine. The healthcare act of the Obama administration was going to see to that. Almost 10 years later, I'm still waiting. Most health insurances companies don't pay for complementary medicine, but if you want surgery or drugs, you have coverage. We have to start seeing change. So many people could benefit from integrating the medicines, it only makes sense. Most recently there are discussions about Medicare starting to pay for acupuncture for pain-related conditions and to ease the opioid crisis we are experiencing in 2019. I'm hoping that the saying "When pigs fly!" comes true soon. For people with asthma and allergies, the treatments haven't changed in years and you are stuck in the sick care paradigm and you're getting sicker. You decide. Do you want Healthcare to maintain your health or do you want to only get care when you are already sick or have a disease diagnosis? It's up to you.

What are your feelings about this topic? Make your notes here:

Chapter 5

What is Traditional Chinese Medicine (TCM)?

The National Center for Complementary and Integrative Health (NIH) defines TCM as an ancient medicine that uses various mind-body practices such as acupuncture, moxibustion, herbal medicine, tuina (Chinese massage) dietary therapy, qi gong, and Tai Chi to treat or prevent health problems. In the USA people use TCM primarily as a complementary health approach. It has become more popular in the last 10 years and there are some hospitals in major cities which are starting to integrate Chinese Medicine into their facilities, but it is not yet mainstream.

Brief History of Acupuncture and Chinese Medicine

Discoveries of ancient documents and scrolls believed to be more than 4000 years old are the first records known in China that support the origins of acupuncture, moxibustion, and herbal medicine practice.

(Chinese Acupuncture and Moxibustion, Page 1 to 11)

Dr. Shen Nong is believed to be the father of herbal medicine. It is said that he tasted hundreds of plants in a day and that he poisoned himself more than seventy times to understand how plants work on the human body.

(Basic Theory of Chinese Medicine Page 1)

Emperor Huangdi's internal classic on TCM was written in the 3rd century B.C. and still has application today. Dr. Fu Xi described stone needles, called bian stone, as the first acupuncture needles. (Basic Concept of Chinese medicine Page 1 to 11)

During the five dynasty periods from 907 to 1368, printing was used to disseminate information on Chinese Medicine and Pharmacology. Today we still see advancements in acupuncture and Chinese medicine with China leading the research, not only in Chinese medicine but with essential oils too. (PubMed)

To understand disease and treatments of disease in ancient times physicians looked for the root causes of disease. This concept continues today with the practice of holistic medicine. Western physicians in modern society look for symptoms and then prescribe drugs.

Main Concepts in Chinese Medicine

Yin and Yang

"Yin and Yang are the laws of heaven and earth, the great framework of everything."

(Chapter 15 of the book on Plain Questions)

49

Every living thing is composed of Yin and Yang. Yin and Yang cannot exist without each other and during life, it is a constant balancing act. Yin is cold, night and female. Yang is hot, day and male. Too much of one can lead to disease or illness and too little can result in death.

Qi

Qi is the essential substance of the human body that affects the organs of the body. I like to think of it as the life force of the body-vital energy. Qi is the commander of the blood. Blood is the mother of Qi. Qi is believed to connect the mind, body, and spirit of a person.

Blood

Blood is a red liquid that circulates in the body. It is a vital nutrient of the body. Blood cannot be separated from Qi. Blood is Yin in nature.

Body Fluids

Body fluids are normal fluids in the body. Examples are saliva, intestinal and gastric juices, sweat, urine, and tears. Qi is different than body fluids but connected. Circulation of Qi is needed to circulate body fluids. These fluids are formed from food and water after digestion and absorption through the spleen and the stomach.

Meridians

Meridians are responsible for the circulation of Qi and Blood throughout the body. The body consists of twelve main meridians that connect internally and externally to the organs, joints, limbs and other tissues of the body. The circulation of the Qi through the Meridians has a cyclical flow. Once stimulated it takes 30 minutes to circulate Qi throughout the body.

Zang Fu

This is the general term for the internal organs of the body. The Zang organs are the lungs, heart, spleen, kidneys, liver, and pericardium. Zang organs manufacture and store essential substances like Qi, Blood, and fluids. The Fu organs are the gall bladder, stomach, small intestine, large intestine, bladder, and triple energizer. The Fu organs receive and digest food.

Acupuncture Points

Acupuncture points are the specific sites on the body through which, it is believed, that the Qi of the organs is transported to the body surface. It takes approximately thirty minutes to circulate the Qi throughout the organs once an acupuncture point is stimulated. There are over 361 acupuncture points on the body that can be used to treat disorders of the body. Application of essential oils, electrical stimulation, or massage to specific acupuncture points can enhance the acupuncture treatment or stimulate the points in the absence of needles and can be done at home once the correct points are identified.

Some Important Acupuncture Points

When treating asthma and allergies, the following points can be very effective in improving respiratory function and overall wellness. Cun is one inch in Chinese.

Chinese Name-Location-Indications

San Yin Jiao- Spleen-6; this point is located on the medial lower leg. This point treats abdomen pain, diarrhea, bleeding uterus, hernia, and muscle atrophy.

Zu San Li- Stomach-36; this point is located on the lateral leg 3 cun below the knee. This point treats gastric pain, vomiting, hiccups, abdomen distention, and diarrhea.

Tai Chong- Liver-3; this point is located between the big toe and second toe 2 cun below the web. This point treats insomnia, dizziness, ankle pain, hypochondria, abdomen, eye, head, hernia, urine retention, and epilepsy.

Hegu- Large Intestine 4; this point is located between the thumb and second finger at the end of the crease. This point treats neck pain, head, eye, teeth, nasal obstruction, and deafness, swelling of face, weakness of limbs, sore throat, and fever.

Liegue- Lung 7; this point is located on the arm just above the base of the thumb. This point treats breathing issues, headache, neck stiffness, cough, sore throat, and pain.

Feishu- Bladder 13; this point is the back Shu point of the lungs. This point is located on the neck at the C7 level. This point treats asthma, cough, and stiffness of the back.

Feng Chi- Gallbladder 20; this wind point is located on the neck just below the skull. This point treats the common cold, headache, dizziness, pain, runny mucus and stiffness in the neck.

Shenman- HT 7; this point is located on the lateral wrist. This point treats cardiac pain, irritability, insomnia, fever, and sensation in palms.

Jiao Xin- K8; this point is located on the medial leg 2 cun above the ankle bone. This point treats irregular menstruation, uterine bleeding, prolapse, pain and swelling of the testis, back pain and tonifies the kidney.

Yangling Quan- GB 34; this point is located on the lateral leg just below the junction of the tibia and fibula. This point treats tendons, weakness, numbness, pain in lower extremities, swelling and pain of the knee, hypochondriac, pain, vomiting, and bitter taste in the mouth.

Bai Hui- DU 20; this point is located directly on top of the head. This point treats headache, coma, mental disorders, prolapse of uterus and rectum, and spreads Qi to over 100 points in the body.

Houxi-SI 3; this point is located on the ulnar border of the hand. This point treats pain, neck stiffness, tinnitus, deafness, sore throat lumbar strain, and numbness in fingers.

Yin Tang- This is an extra point between the eyes. This point treats headache, sinus congestion, and is a happy point for well-being.

Diagnosis and Treatment of Disease

Diagnosis and treatment of disease are analyzed through a process called a Pattern of Syndrome Differentiation. Syndrome Differentiation looks for the root cause of disease and is the main function of Chinese medicine. Once a person's pattern is determined, the doctor will treat the person with a variety of modalities, such as acupuncture, moxibustion, gua sha, laser, herbal medicine and/or essential oils. There are other diagnostic methods, each having its own limitations and benefits, but I use Syndrome Differentiation in my clinic. If you are ready to make your healthcare a priority, Chinese medicine is right for you! Chinese medicine may seem complex due to the unfamiliar terms, but if you think about health as a balance between you and nature, you will start to understand when your body tells you something is out of balance, and you will know how to respond with Chinese medicine.

Chapter 6

Chinese Medicine Modalities

How Chinese Medicine can help Asthma and Allergies

Asthma is a condition where the tubes leading to the lungs reacts to exterior pathogens like smoke, dust, dust mites, chemicals, pollen, molds, foods, and pet dander. The lungs react to the exposure to the pathogen and swell and produce phlegm, causing coughing, wheezing and breathing problems. This leads to the narrowing of the bronchial tubes. When this occurs, your body produces antibodies called IGG and IGE. Research suggests that exposure to second-hand smoke and a family history of asthma could be a contributing factor in developing asthma. No one knows why some people develop asthma and some don't, but the root cause is inflammation leading to changes in the body. Asthma is closely linked to allergies. The Center for Disease Control (CDC) reports that as of 2016 approximately 8.3 % of the US population, or 26 million people, have been diagnosed with asthma. Additionally, 7.6 million people are also reported to have respiratory allergy problems, an increase from approximately 5 million in 2003 according to the CDC prevention report from that year. Surprisingly the treatments for allergies and asthma have not changed significantly in all those years. There is a new class of drugs available now that are called biologics, but still, the drug companies claim that asthma cannot be cured. And by the way, many of the drugs prescribed for asthma suppress the body's responses so that the chance of death is much higher while on these drugs. Statistics on asthma prevalence, activity limitation, days of work or school lost, rescue and control medication use, asthma self-management education, physician visits, hospital emergency visits, hospitalizations due to asthma, and deaths due to asthma are tracked by the National Center for Health Statistics (NCHS) surveys and the Vital Statistics System. The treatments for allergies and asthma by western doctors include prescription of steroids, reuse inhalers, leukotriene receptor inhibitor meds, prednisone, allergy shots, and over the counter meds like Benadryl. Also, the new biologic drugs are injected. The patient package inserts that come with the medicines are very important to read prior to agreeing to take the meds. This rarely happens though. I never read them until I began to have rashes, itchy skin, dark circles under my eyes, coughing, and raspy throat and wasn't feeling better. The day I quit taking the allergy shots was my first step to healing my body. The solutions in those shots made me feel sicker and never did anything to stop my constant sinus infections, coughing, or the side effects of the meds. In fact, a review of the patient package inserts list many of the symptoms I was feeling.

Things to do:

- Write down all your symptoms

- Write down all the meds you are taking

- Read all the Patient Package Inserts (PPI) for the meds you are taking

- List all your side effects

Do you see any connection between your symptoms and side effects listed in the PPI of the meds your taking?

Things that can trigger Asthma:

- Medicines like aspirin and beta blockers (used to treat high blood pressure)
- Sulfites in foods (used as a preservative)
- Infections
- GERD (gastroesophageal reflux)

Questions:

- Do you catch colds often? If so, how long do they last?

- Do you have a family history of asthma and allergies?

- Were you ever exposed to second-hand smoke?

- Are you taking any pharmaceuticals, homeopathic drugs or supplements?

- Do you experience coughing, wheezing, sneezing, chest discomfort or tightness, shortness of breath? If so when does this happen? Can you relate it to anything?

Write your answers below:

Many symptoms can be worse at night with asthma. The explanation for this is not really understood fully but the liver, which is the biggest organ in the body, is believed to be less active at night and therefore influences other organs to be less active which then causes a deficiency in the body. Asthma and allergies are more common in women than men as adults, but boys suffer from asthma more in childhood. This can be explained by the changes in hormone levels that happen in women during menstrual cycles, pregnancy, and menopause. Allergy testing and food sensitivity testing is a very important part of the process. At Alternative Natural Healthcare, we use gold standard testing companies to help us identify your sensitivities. We all have read about food and supplements that are good for you, but until you are tested you don't know what is more harmful than good for you. I had never eaten mung beans before I lived in Asia. Recently I was food tested and have a 2 plus sensitivity to mung beans, which is a frequently prescribed food for asthma. With advancements in testing, we are seeing a lot of new information pop up that is helpful for understanding a person's future course of treatment. Specifically, genetic testing is showing us what pharmaceuticals could benefit you if you need to take any drug, and which ones never to take because of your genetic profile. It should be mandatory that all doctors test a patient before prescribing drugs, but this doesn't happen in allopathic medicine. You need to find a complementary practitioner to do this. The treatments in allopathic medicine for allergies have not changed much and the most prescribed methods are allergy shots. Putting more toxicity into your body with the hope your immune system will improve is counterproductive to me. Our goal at Alternative Natural Healthcare is to help you boost your immune system naturally, not bog it down with vaccinations and other synthetic drugs and preservatives that have a negative effect on the body. They also can be linked to autoimmune diseases and other debilitating diseases like paralysis, shingles, measles, and death. Instead of suppressing symptoms and taking a chance of a bad outcome, why not work on boosting your immune system naturally? A new way of thinking, that's not so new. Allergic rhinitis is a common complaint seen in the clinic. Symptoms can be itching in the nose or throat, sneezing, mucus production, shortness of breath, weak voice, white coating appearing on the tongue, stuffiness or congestion in the head and nose. This can all be caused by exposure to exterior pathogens and due to the lung, kidney, and spleen being deficient in their energy Qi, your body then becomes sensitive to the exposure. Just being exposed to cold air alone could have a negative effect on the body if your Qi isn't strong. Sneezing is always the first sign that your body is being attacked by a pathogen and very frequently you will become ill after sneezing begins. Sneezing is also the last symptom you should have when getting over an attack. Warming the body thru moxa (this is a new word, what is it??) and diet is very important in aiding the body to recovery. Many people don't even realize they are very cold when they come to the clinic because they have had a disease for a very long time and have become accustomed to being cold. Once they begin to tonify the body, they begin to feel better. They are always surprised at how lying under a heat lamp can rejuvenate them. Herbal medicine can also help warm and reset the body. Eating foods that grow during each season would be the best way to start tonifying your body, but in today's world, all foods are available all the time making this very hard. Many people have the same foods every day all year long, leading to food sensitivities. If you can start to grow some of your food and greens and start juicing seasonal foods, you will feel better faster.

Microsystems

The hands, feet, and ears are considered microsystems. This means that the organs of the body are represented in different positions on the hand, feet, and ears. Treatment of microsystems is an effective and powerful way to treat a person's pattern of differentiation. See **Modern Essentials, The Complete Guide to the Use of Therapeutic Essential Oils** for charts on the hands, feet, and ears. (8th edition, pages 18-20) This picture shows the organs of the body represented in the foot. Stimulation of these areas with acupuncture, massage or just

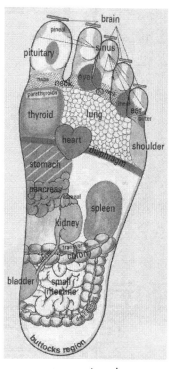

applying an essential oil to the areas you want to stimulate can help relieve your symptoms. Breathlessness or Chuan Zheng in Chinese is a condition where your breathing is very fast and shallow. Many people have difficulty inhaling the breath and keep their mouth open to breathe. Lying down may make breathing worse. This is very common with asthma. In

Chinese medicine, this is caused by the lung Qi's failure to descend. This can be caused by phlegm obstructing the lungs, exposure to excessive wind or cold or heat in the lungs. Deficiencies of the kidney and lungs channels are also factors in the Qi failing to descend. People that are under a lot of stress, have a chronic illness or eat improper diets can make the deficiencies even worse. Your pattern of deficiency can be determined by your Acupuncture Physician and a diagnosis of syndrome differentiation can be made. You may have the excess syndrome, and focusing on treating the lungs is of the utmost importance when trying to get rid of phlegm and expelling pathogens. If you have a deficiency syndrome treating both the kidney and lungs would be the preferred treatment. Some people can have a deficiency with excess, so a careful diagnosis must be made. Depending on your diagnosis you may need herbal medicine in conjunction with your acupuncture treatments. Herbal medicines are very helpful and are only taken until the symptoms disappear. This is not a lifetime commitment. Most herbal medicines are not that expensive and work fairly quickly. Knowing how to protect yourself from future pathogenic attacks is important for keeping your body healthy going forward. My grandmother always wanted me to keep my head warm with a scarf, to avoid being out in wind and to eat warm food in winter. I never understood at the time, but it really makes sense to modify your lifestyle according to the time of year. If you are mindful of the season changes you can begin to manage your health in a positive way.

ACUPUNCTURE: WHAT IS IT?

Acupuncture is a form of healthcare that has a 5000-year history. This is done by inserting needles at certain points on the body. Heat lamps or Avazzia micro current can be used to enhance the effectiveness of the needles. Laser therapy and injection therapy can also be used at certain points in the body.

HOW DOES ACUPUNCTURE WORK?

I am always asked this question, and I always say yes it works. You do not need to be a believer to make it work. Insertion of needles in acupuncture points triggers the brain to release certain chemicals and hormones in the body that are directed to the area of discomfort, pain or malfunction. Thus, stimulating the body to begin to heal itself. Increases of blood flow and circulation are seen too.

HOW CAN I USE ACUPUNCTURE FOR MY HEALTH CONDITIONS?

Acupuncture can be used for:

- Promotion of health and well-being.

- Prevention of illness.
- Treatment of various medical conditions.

Though acupuncture is often used for pain control, An Acupuncture Physician, can provide you lifestyle, dietary and supplement recommendations that will enhance your acupuncture treatments. Acupuncture can be used alone or in combination with other treatment forms for many medical disorders.

HOW MANY TREATMENTS WILL I NEED?

The number of treatments required vary depending on the person and the complaint. That being said I recommend that every new patient receive ten (10) treatments to start and then their case be evaluated to determine if more treatment is needed. I always recommend getting acupuncture when the seasons change and whenever you are sick or have a health concern.

Acupuncture is very effective in treating respiratory diseases and allergies. Once the root cause of the respiratory problem is identified the patient should get results in a short period of time. Each treatment plan is different and times for treatment vary.

Gua Sha or Scraping Therapy

Gua Sha or Scraping therapy is an ancient Chinese medicine method used to treat respiratory ailments. It is performed using a tool made from the horn of a buffalo. The tool is pressed on the skin and light to medium pressure is used to scrape across the skin. This creates an irritation on the skin leaving petechia. This will allow the blood to come to the top of the skin, increasing blood flow and circulation. It assists the body to dispose of toxins that might be in the skin, move phlegm out of lungs and aid in recovery from the respiratory attack. See chapter 7 for a photo of a patient receiving Gua Sha. The treatment is well tolerated and looks worse than it is. Patients will have light bruising for a few days following therapy. It is recommended that the patient drink plenty of hot liquids following this therapy. Patients that have a weak constitution, body rashes, or haven't eaten should not get Gua Sha. Gua Sha is a strong treatment that moves a lot of Qi blood and lymph and could cause fatigue in the person receiving the treatment. Your acupuncture physician will be able to determine if it is right for you.

Cupping

Cupping is another ancient Chinese therapy that is very effective in treating respiratory diseases as well as pain issues. Glass, bamboo or plastic cups are applied to the skin with either a pump or flash fire technique and remain in place for approximately 15-20 minutes. The cups can also be moved around once placed to stimulate the whole channel they are on. This therapy like Gua Sha produces petechia and leaves a round shaped bruise on the skin. The goal with cupping is to restore the normal blood flow and circulation to the areas being treated and restore the area's normal function. See Chapter 7 for a photo of the type of cups commonly used in treatment. Cupping does not hurt at all when done properly.

Herbal Medicine

Restoring the body to homeostasis is the goal in Chinese medicine. Pharmaceuticals can stop the pain and kill bacteria, but they cannot strengthen the body, or stop the disease from progressing. They also have unwanted side effects and can damage organs like kidneys and stomach, cause nerve damage, and can cause nervous system disorders. If you never cure the root cause of disease you will be taking pharmaceuticals for life. Hippocrates said around 480 BC, "Let your food be your medicine and your medicine be your food". We are so far from that idea in today's lifestyles that it is no wonder that we see so many inflammatory diseases. Chinese herbal medicines are decocted from ginger, tangerine, apricot seeds, roots leaves, stems, bark, and flowers. Almost any part of a plant can be used for something. They are almost always combined together with more than one different herb to provide the delicate balance needed to treat disease while avoiding side effects. Understanding the properties of herbal medicines are important when prescribing them to treat asthma and allergies. If your pattern of differentiation is a cold disease, herbs that are warm or hot in the property must be selected. Examples of warm or hot herbal medicines are ginger, cinnamon, clove, oregano, and thyme. The peel from the tangerine fruit is commonly used to treat airway constriction and control asthma. Boiling water with the rinds of the fruit makes a very fragrant tea that is enjoyable to drink and has many health benefits. This tea contains vitamin C and vitamin B which help cellular energy. The apricot seed is another bitter, slightly warm herb that helps stop coughing and eases difficult breathing. Perilla fruit is often served with sushi and used to treat food poisoning. Perilla fruit is also used to increase Qi to remove phlegm from the lungs. It's warm acrid properties help transform phlegm by drying the fluid. There are many Chinese herbs and formulas used for asthma and allergies. Your Chinese medicine doctor will know what is right for you. The formulas can come in pills, capsules, liquid or injection form.

Diet

In addition to using herbs to control asthma and allergies, diet is a very important factor. There are many foods that have reported effects beneficial to people that have asthma and allergies, but I recommend food sensitivity testing before a diet is suggested.

Things to start doing before you are tested:

- Stop drinking iced beverages
- Do not smoke
- Do not drink alcohol
- Do not overeat

- Eat neutral foods and avoid spicy foods

- Do not eat greasy foods

- Reduce sugar and salt intake

Exercise, Medical Qi Gong

Exercise

Chinese medicine incorporates a series of body movements, breathing, and massage. These are believed to help balance the Yin and Yang and restore the body to homeostasis. This is done with an exercise called medical Qi Gong. This can be done sitting in a chair, standing or laying down. A plan can be devised for each person individually, based on their specific needs. Sitting too much is very harmful to your body. You must get up and move around for at least 10-15 mins per hour. Standing, stretching, walking and swimming can help restore one's vitality very quickly when you get in a habit of doing something every day. If you have a desk job you need to modify your work station to allow for a standing desk. You can also do small circular movements with your feet ankles and legs while at your desk. A protocol based on your syndrome differentiation will be prescribed for you so that you can do it at home daily.

Chapter 7

Photo Gallery

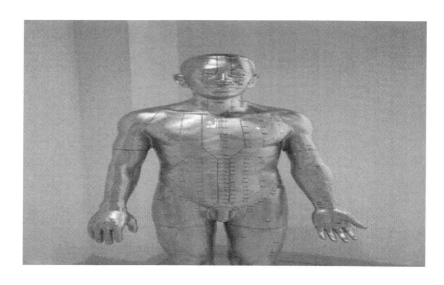

Acupuncture man is a very famous model showing all the acupuncture points identified on the human body. There are over 361 points on the body, but only a few points are chosen for each treatment. The points on the neck, upper back and on the arms are very effective for treating asthma and allergies.

BODY MERIDIANS

Governing Vessel
Conception Vessel
Small Intestine Meridian
Stomach Meridian
Spleen Meridian
Lung Meridian
Heart Meridian
Bladder Meridian
Kidney Meridian
Liver Meridian
Large Intestine Meridian
Pericardium Meridian
Triple Warmer Meridian
Gall Bladder Meridian

This picture shows the meridians of the body and how they travel. The Qi of the body circulates thru these meridians and are connected to each other in a complex system of roots and branches.

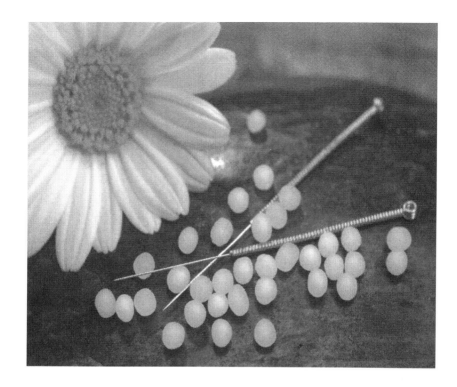

Acupuncture needles come in all sizes and lengths. The most common sizes used in the clinic are 1 and 1 ½ inch long and only 40 gauge. Ear acupuncture needles are a ½ inch long and 40 gauge. All needles are only used 1 time and come in sterilized packs. Homeopathic remedies are usually in pill form as small balls showed above or tablets.

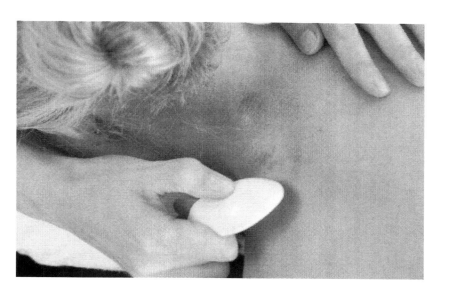

Scraping therapy is a very effective therapy for treating allergies and asthma. The skin is scraped with a device made from a buffalo horn. This causes petechia to form releasing pathogens from under the skin. It looks worse than it is! Most people report the treatment is very tolerable and that they feel relief from their symptoms 1-2 days after treatment.

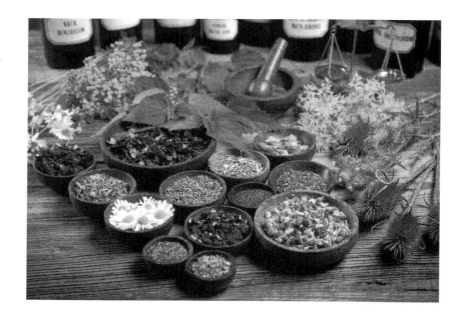

Chinese herbal medicines are made from flowers, roots, stems, and leaves of plants. The medicines are an important part of the treatment plan that is determined from your diagnosis.

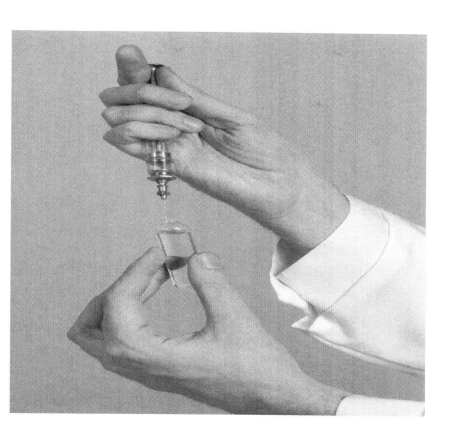

Acupuncture Injection Therapy with homeopathic medicines is an effective treatment for asthma and allergies. Specific homeopathic medicines are injected into acupuncture points to target detox, repair, and rejuvenation.

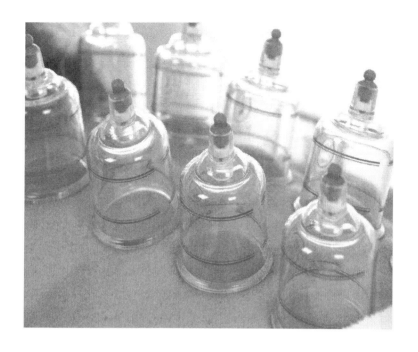

Cupping is done with either plastic, silicone or glass cups. They are attached to the body by suction and then moved around the body. This causes blood to move into the muscle tissue, increasing circulation and blood flow to the area treated. Bruising can happen during cupping, but it is not dangerous.

Chapter 8

Acupuncture Injection Therapy

Acupuncture Point Injection, or Acupoint Injection Therapy (AIT), is an integrative therapy that blends the best of Chinese medicine with conventional and homeopathic medicine. Employing this technique, an AIT certified acupuncture physician injects natural therapeutic substances, such as homeopathic remedies or vitamins, into acupuncture points specific to your wellness needs. By stimulating powerful acupuncture points with proven natural substances, we can affect the body on a deeper level and create a healing climate. AIT is particularly effective for the resolution of acute and chronic pain in the body, particularly in the shoulder, back, knee, and neck. We also use AIT techniques in many of our weight loss protocols, Cosmetic Acupuncture programs, and even our B-12 injections. Sometimes referred to as "bio puncture," AIT earned well-deserved attention in early 2011 and again in 2014 when Dr. Mehmet Oz featured the therapy on his television show. In order to utilize AIT as a therapy, licensed acupuncture physicians in Florida must complete additional didactic and clinical training beyond their traditional education. Additional 60-hour certification in AIT must be earned in order to practice this technique. Florida administrative law allows property trained acupuncture physicians to provide AIT pursuant to the following rule:

64B1-4.012 Acupoint Injection Therapies.

"Effective March 1, 2002, adjunctive therapies shall include acupoint injection therapy which shall mean the injection of herbs, homeopathic, and other nutritional supplements in the form of sterile substances into acupuncture points by means of hypodermic needles but not intravenous therapy to promote, maintain, and restore health; for pain management and palliative care; for acupuncture anesthesia; and to prevent disease." Not all acupuncturists can perform AIT and not all states allow AIT. You should check with your individual state for allowed services. The AIT protocols used for the treatment of asthma and allergies are determined for each patient after a complete evaluation. The purest high-quality homeopathic medicine is used at Alternative Natural Healthcare. It can be injected for faster results or pills can be prescribed. Treating asthma or allergy patients that do not like acupuncture needles may prefer this method of treatment. Using the lung points and tonifying points with AIT are very helpful in restoring homeostasis and eliminating the need for western drugs.

Homeopathy, or Homeopathic Medicine

Dr Samuel Hahnemann (1755-1843) was a practitioner and a medical translator. His work as a translator exposed him to a vast range of concepts, observations and approaches. He noted in some of the documents a recurring theme of how low dose of a substance, at times helped to resolve the ailment. He started to experiment with this concept and in many instances, saw favorable results. His research extended not just to pathogens (the beginning of low dose immune therapy, vaccines), but also other substances. The term "Like cures Like" comes from Hippocrates (460-377 BC), it is a guiding homeopathic principle. The word homeopathy comes from Greek through Latin which literally means "like disease". Its comes from the observations of cases where a diluted or low dose of the substance which causes the issues helps to resolve it. These concepts became the base of what is now used for allergies and vaccines. He recorded his meticulous work in his Materia Medicas. Through his work he discovered that a sequential dilution process where a substance is diluted down to the desired concentration in steps of 1 part in 10 (noted as X or D dilutions) or 1 part in 100 (C dilutions) yielded better results over a direct dilution to the desired concentration, meaning 1 part per million (PPM) can either be made by 1 part in a million (now the allopathic standard) or 1 part in 10 done is 6 sequential steps noted as a 6X or D6 or 1 part in 100 done in 3 sequential steps noted as 3C. All these preparation methods come to 1 PPM. A difference in the preparation method is for a homeopathic the mixing process is done by a vigorous shaking process where the container is

banged against a hard surface during each step of the diluting process while the straight dilution process is often stirred in some fashion. Further work recognized that each concentration has a different effect on the subject. Some dilutions of the substance help to stimulate, others regulate, while others sedate. A number of other practitioners complemented his work by performing their own studies and writing them up in Materia Medicas, case studies, articles, and papers. A Materia Medica description of a substance encompasses observations of the physical, physiological, psychological, emotional, neurological, endocrine, symptomatic, thematic and other factors of the entire scope of a substance's action, many include interactions, complementary substances and ones to avoid. Classical homeopaths follow in this tradition and keep expanding the wealth of knowledge. As for the government guidance, the Homeopathic Pharmacopoeia of the United States has been in continuous publication since 1897, when it was first published by the Committee on Pharmacy of the American Institute of Homeopathy. Prior to that, pharmacopoeias had been published by Boericke and Tafel (1882) and Jahr (1841). Canada, England, France, Germany, Europe, India, Australia and a number of other countries all have a homeopathic pharmacopeia as part of their regulations. These pharmacopeias provide government standards and regulations for homeopathic cGMP's, they are as demanding as those for drugs. Materia Medicas formed the founding evidence base for the standards. A homeopathic is the first dilution the government deems safe for human consumption, meaning if you juice an apple, the government deems apple juice safe for human consumption at this concentration, the only thing which makes a homeopathic different is that the juice needs to be shaken. As Bond would say: "Shaken, not stirred.", so yes, his Martinis have a homeopathic aspect to them. If the first safe concentration is a part in a 1,000 then a 3X or D3 is first concentration used, a part per million or PPM is a 6X/D6 or 3C dilution. At least 95% of all homeopathic's are in the physical range, easily detectable. I use Viatrexx homeopathic medicines because they specialize in targeted formulas which encompass nano or physiological concentration of metabolic factors and supporting or scaffolding substances to enhance the desired action of the formula (immune, repair/anti-aging, detox/drainage,). They also use a proprietary homeopathic method which mimics the heart beat in order to achieve better quality messenger molecule activated molecules.

Dr. Brown's Top Ten Remedies

1. Stomach Discomfort

2. Vomiting

3. Urinary Tract Infection

4. Pain

5. Quit Smoking

6. High Blood Pressure

7. Diabetes

8. Hormone Imbalance

9. Uplifting Mood

10. Scar Aid

1 Stomach Discomfort

As we age, one of the most important functions of the body is in maintaining healthy digestion. Diseases of the stomach are seen with changes in functions of receiving, digesting and elimination of food. This function can be easy impaired by eating greasy foods, foods that are too cold, eating junk foods, eating too late at night and many other factors. Signs of burping, belching, stomachache, gas, hiccups, vomiting, or bloating can indicate dysfunction. A determination by an acupuncture physician to determine whether there is a deficiency or excess in the stomach channel is important. Also looking to see if a person is cold or hot or whether food is being retained are factors to consider.

Ginger- Sheng Jiang is fresh ginger with warm acrid and spicy properties that warm the spleen and stomach. It can be used to warm the stomach and stop vomiting, warm the lungs to stop cough and assist the body to eliminate toxins and disperse the attack of a pathogen. Ginger essential oil is approximately 90% sesquiterpenes which are antiseptic, warming, and stimulating. Applying ginger directly to the abdomen or bottom of the feet can be quite effective in easing discomfort and restoring the stomach to homeostasis.

Peppermint- Bo He, or menthol, is an important Chinese herbal medicine. Menthan Piperita is approximately 45% menthol with analgesic, antibacterial anti-inflammatory, antiviral and invigorating properties. Peppermint is in the exterior reliving category of Chinese medicine and if used topically on the neck and head, it relieves pain and is believed to release pathogens in the superficial layers of the skin.

Cardamom– Doukou in Chinese is an essential oil from the ginger family. It has anti-inflammatory, antiseptic, decongestant and anti-bacterial properties. It can be taken internally or applied to acupuncture or reflex points.

Lemon–Essential oils of lemon come from the rind of the fruit. Lemon is very fragrant and uplifting. From the citrus family, the lemon essential oil is approximately 90% monoterpenes, giving it anti-fungal, anti-cancer, antiviral and antiseptic properties.

2 Vomiting

Prepare a tea by mixing 2 drops of ginger essential oil, 2 drops of lemon essential oil, and 1 drop of peppermint in hot water and sip slowly. A teaspoon of honey can be added. Smelling the ginger essential oil from the bottle for 1-2 minutes could ease the urge to vomit. Topical application of cardamom just below the breast bone and in the belly button with a warm compress for 30 minutes prior to drinking this tea could also ease symptoms. This is a very common complaint with people suffering from respiratory problems because the lung Qi is so weak it causes the reverse of its function.

Stimulation of the Stomach 36, or Zu San Li. This point is located three (3) finger widths below the outer eye of the knee. This is a very powerful power point that can be used to stimulate the stomach organ. By tapping strongly on this point for 10 times it is believed that you can create a response in the body stronger than eating chicken soup when ill.

3 UTI -Urinary Tract Infections

As we age UTIs are seen more frequently. One main reason is that the bladder does not empty completely and a bacterium starts to grow. Another factor is the nerve function that signals your bladder

is full declines and the notice is not made. I always advise my patients to try to urinate completely. You can do this by trying to squeeze out more urine after you think you are done urinating and by urinating frequently. Take your time when urinating and don't rush. In Chinese medicine, UTIs fall into the category of painful urinary syndromes. Symptoms can be pain upon urination, frequent urination, difficult or sporadic urination, and urgency. Juniper Berry is a well-known cleaner, detoxifier, antispasmodic, antiseptic, stimulant and tonic. It is distilled from the berries of the cypress tree. It works well with Geranium, and Tangerine to promote detoxification. Juniper Berry Essential oil applied to the lower abdomen and kidney areas with a warm compress is recommended as well as making a Juniper Berry tea. Use 2-4 drops of Juniper Berry in hot water and sip one to two cups 3 times a day until the problem resolves itself. Application of 2 drops of Juniper Berry, 2 drops of Tangerine and 1 drop of Geranium to the bottom of your feet especially in the kidney area may also be effective in eliminating symptoms.

Acupuncture to the Ren 3 Point, Zhong Ji; Spleen 9, Yin Ling Quan, and Bladder 28, Pang Guan Shu can help unblock the obstructions and promote the elimination of the pathogen.

4 Pain

Pain, whether in the head, neck, back, knees, arms, legs or hands, can be an aggravating and debilitating life-altering condition. In Chinese medicine, it is believed that pain is due to

Qi and blood stagnation in the body. This can happen from injury, illness, arthritis, or other dysfunctions in the body. The primary cause for pain in the body, besides external pathogens that attack the body, is the deficiency of the kidney function. This doesn't mean your kidney is failing but in Chinese medicine, the kidney is believed to be the source of the original Yin and Yang of the body. As we age the energy of the kidney is in decline. We need to constantly find ways to tonify this function.

This can be done by using tonifying herbs and regular acupuncture treatments to treat the local pain areas as well as focusing on tonifying and warming the kidneys. Application of essential oils to the areas of concern can help warm the area and increase blood flow and circulation. My favorites are Fir oils, like Siberian Fir or White Fir, Wintergreen, Lemongrass, Birch, and Blue Tansy. There are pain blends, and massage blends that are available too. I never recommend using ice for more than a few days after an injury or the start of pain in an area. Ice freezes the area causing damage to the tissue and constricts blood flow. Using steam heat is a better idea as it increases blood flow and circulation, which can stop the pain.

Pain Relief at Home - Using Avazzia micro stimulation is also very beneficial in treating pain. Pain relief at home is now available in both over-the-counter and prescription relief options. They are handheld, drug free, non-surgical, non-invasive microcurrent devices that are safe and easy to use.

Avazzia prescription devices are FDA cleared for symptomatic relief and management of chronic, intractable pain, and adjunctive treatment in the management of post-surgical and post traumatic pain. Avazzia over-the-counter devices are FDA cleared for the temporary relief of pain associated with sore and aching muscles in the shoulder, waist, back, back of neck, upper extremities (arm), and lower extremities (leg) due to strain from exercise or normal household work activities. No prescription required. People have found tremendous relief of pain with both prescription devices and over the counter devices with the following: Headaches, Chronic Fatigue, Abdominal, Rheumatoid Arthritis, Neuropathy, Scar Tissue, TMJ, Carpal Tunnel, Scoliosis, Back, Wounds, Whiplash, Gas, Diarrhea, Constipation, Anxiety, Fibromyalgia, MS, Tendons, Ligaments, Joints, Shingles, Burns. The Avazzia technology works differently than most TENS units because they have a High-Speed Microprocessor that establishes a cybernetic loop between the BEST (Bio-Electric Stimulation Technology) device and the body. The body's response is measurable, creating information for the loop. When the signal is emitted and penetrates deep into the tissue, the impedance of the tissue modulates the next waveform. The degree of modulation is based upon the changes of the impedance of the skin. This sets up a continually changing interactive bio-loop processing non-repeating signals so your body can't become habitual to it. Eventually, the change in impedance diminishes in significance until a plateau occurs, and most people experience pain relief. The body has an inherent capability of maintaining its own health and function and communicates via micro-currents. Over the centuries, Western medicine has focused on pharmaceutical cures fir illnesses and damaged tissues. Avazzia takes technology that has been known for decades and brings it into the 21st century. Avazzia devices put control of your pain in your hands. A physician or other healthcare provider needs to assess your medical condition and history. Once it is determined, Avazzia is right for you, Avazzia allows you to take control of your health and pain management. The single purchase of an Avazzia device, over its lifetime, is far less than the cost of over-the-counter drugs or prescription drugs and far less than even minimally invasive surgery. For more information, go to www.firstalternativetherapies.com. Use coupon code (off the Meds) for any device and receive $50.00 off.

5 Quit Smoking

Addiction to cigarettes is a global problem. The toxic chemicals used in making cigarettes are very harmful and addictive to the body. Cancer and other harmful respiratory diseases are seen in people who use these products. Quitting can be difficult for many people. Using the NADA protocol, which is a 10-point needling protocol in the ears, along with essential oils, can help support the body when stopping the use of toxic addictive chemicals. Peppermint, Licorice, Clove, and Hyssops are common essential oils and Chinese herbs that can assist in the addiction recovery.

Recipe:

Add the following to one to two cups hot or cold green tea:

2 drops of peppermint

2 drops of licorice

2 drops of Hyssop

Drink 2 -3 times a day.

Use Clove on the back of the tongue to help with cravings. Clove is hot so use 1 drop on a Q-tip and place on the back on the tongue.

6 High Blood Pressure (HBP)

Hypertension is the same thing as high blood pressure. It happens when the blood is moving thru the arteries at a high speed. This can cause weakness in the vessels if left untreated. HBP is often undiagnosed for many years; however, some people are aware of when their pressure is high. Dizziness, headaches, and flushing in the face can be seen, indicating an HBP issue. Untreated HBP can lead to heart issues, strokes or even death. Healthy function of blood pressure is essential for a healthy body. Getting your blood pressure checked at your doctor's office annually is a good idea to establish baseline numbers for yourself. Many people now are purchasing home units to check their blood pressure. You can also go to most pharmacies and find a machine to check your pressure. Everyone has different pressures and it can change very quickly. You need to have a series of readings or do blood pressure monitoring to know for sure what your blood pressure does throughout the day. Blood pressure can change due to stress, improper diet or kidney essence deficiency. The American Heart Association sets guidelines for blood pressure shown in the chart below:

BLOOD PRESSURE CATEGORY	SYSTOLIC mm Hg (upper number)		DIASTOLIC mm Hg (lower number)
NORMAL	LESS THAN 120	and	LESS THAN 80
ELEVATED	120 – 129	and	LESS THAN 80
HIGH BLOOD PRESSURE (HYPERTENSION) STAGE 1	130 – 139	or	80 – 89
HIGH BLOOD PRESSURE (HYPERTENSION) STAGE 2	140 OR HIGHER	or	90 OR HIGHER
HYPERTENSIVE CRISIS (consult your doctor immediately)	HIGHER THAN 180	and/or	HIGHER THAN 120

If your blood pressure is in stage one or higher ranges, you should consult with a doctor and start making lifestyle changes like dietary changes and exercise. (Medical Diagnosis and Treatment, Chapter 11, McGraw Medical Online)

Acupuncture combined with essential oils application, diet and exercise have shown to improve blood pressure readings. Ear acupuncture is always used as supportive therapy for high blood pressure, as well as body points GB 20 Fengchi, GB 34 Yang Ling Quan, SP 6 San Yin Jiao, LI 4 Hegu, and St 36 Zu San Li. There are some Chinese herbal medicine formulas for HBP depending on your pattern of differentiation. Determining your pattern of differentiation will determine the correct needling protocols. Essential oils that have shown to aid in reducing HBP are Marjoram, Lemon, Ylang Ylang, and Clary Sage and Lavender. I like to add Marjoram and lemon teas to the diet of people who have HBP. Boil 2 cups of water and add 2-4 drops of Marjoram and 2 drops of Lemon essential oils. If you don't tolerate the taste of essential oils, you can rub the oils directly on the bottom of your feet. The biggest pores in the body are there and facilitate fast absorption of the oils. This way you don't lose any of the oils thru the first pass effect of the kidney and liver filtering out what is taken into the body. Low blood pressure can be a concern too. This can cause dizziness and heart palpitations. Eating high-quality sea salt may help with this issue. Stay away from iodized salts as they are nothing but synthetic chemicals that are not well tolerated by the body. Many pharmaceuticals have a side effect of lowering blood pressure and causing dizziness. Check the patient package insert for the drugs you are prescribed. If you experience these side effects report them to your doctor immediately.

7 Diabetes

Diabetes, called Shou Ke in Chinese medicine, is considered a thirsting and wasting disorder because of dysfunction in the pancreas and liver. Due to this dysfunction, the body is depleting its vital substances. You may also be taking in excessive amounts of food and water, causing imbalance. Additionally, excessive thirst may be experienced which is not relieved by drinking. This dysfunction can be caused by improper diet, emotional stress, and overexertion. All of these factors cause the underlying problem of driving the body's Yin fluids to deficiency. Determining the root cause and location of the disease is important and a trained acupuncture physician can determine if the upper middle or lower Jiao organs are involved. A combination of essential oils that target the metabolic process in the body is recommended. A combination blend of therapeutic grade essential oils like Grapefruit, Lemon, Peppermint, Ginger and Cinnamon has been used to assist with hunger, and weight control as well as warmth and coolness applied to the stomach. They can also provide emotional support. Acupuncture and herbal therapy are recommended to be combined with essential oil intake.

8 Hormone Imbalance

As we age our hormone production starts to decline. In Chinese medicine, we look at the kidney energy. After age 40 the body energy starts to decline and tonification is needed more frequently to preserve the vitality of the body. Essential oils can be applied to the hands or feet or inhaled to assist the body to produce or maintain its hormone levels. Oils that can help are Clary Sage, Ylang Ylang, Rosemary and Clove. A roller ball of 1-3 different oils can be combined in an FCO fractionated coconut base, and rolled on as needed throughout the day and night. Three drops of each oil in a 10-ml rollerball will work: just add the oil and then fill your rollerball with the fractionated coconut oil up to the neck of the bottle and secure the top.

9 Uplifting Mood

Changes in one's mood can happen very quickly if you are tired, have any changes in hormone levels, are dealing with stress or become ill. My favorite oils for uplifting mood are citrus oils: Orange, Lemon, Bergamot, Lavender, Rosemary, Rose, Sandalwood, Ylang-Ylang, and Geranium. They can have a positive impact on mood. You can choose 1-3 different oils and make a blend, depending on your preferences.

10 Scar Aid

Injury to the skin causes the body to produce fibrous connective tissue that forms to help repair the injured areas. This sometimes leaves uneven or bumpy skin. A simple solution to aid the skin in its healing would be to apply equal parts of Frankincense, Myrrh, and Helichrysum in fractionated coconut oil, topically, until the scar improves. Herbal medicine and essential oils can be used to treat many diseases and illnesses. You can learn to incorporate these home remedies into your daily life very easily and will see improved health. There are classes online and, in my clinic, monthly for your education into these topics.

Chapter 10

Obstacles

As with anything worth accomplishing, it will be hard and there will be ups and downs in changing your lifestyle during your path to recovery. You may feel worse after you decide to stop medications or start a new treatment. This is normal and to be expected. Don't give up. If you have any adverse reactions during your treatment tell your physician and your treatment can be adjusted. Always be honest with all of your physicians. I was in a women's clothing store a few months back and overheard some women talking about just finding a new primary healthcare physician and one of the women said that when she went for the initial exam with the doctor she didn't bother to tell the doctor what bioidentical hormones she was taking. The other women said I understand what you're saying, I didn't tell my doctor that I was seeing an acupuncturist for pain either, because he doesn't approve of complementary healthcare. I was surprised. If you don't have confidence in your doctor, why are you going to them? Why can't you tell your doctor what healthcare you want and deserve? You are the customer. You get to decide. Period. No one else can tell you want to do with your body. Your physician works for you. Don't be afraid to discuss your treatment options and force your doctor to make the change to modern medicine. No longer should you go to a doctor and get a pharmaceutical without asking questions and knowing the risks and benefits. Demand alternatives if you don't like the treatment proposed. You are making lifestyle changes, expect to continue to manage your health for the rest of your life. Follow your complementary healthcare doctors' recommendations. Don't take your herbs once or twice and say it doesn't work. Think about how many years you have had the problems you seek to treat and be realistic. Don't expect health insurance to pay for complementary healthcare services. Most insurance companies do not cover acupuncture, herbal medicines or other modalities from acupuncture physicians unless you have a Cadillac plan. Check with your insurance company so you know in advance what your coverage is. Most acupuncture physicians can give you a superbill that you can submit to your insurance company if they don't do insurance billing. There are Chinese medicine doctors in every state in the USA now. You can locate a board-certified physician thru the NCCAOM website by searching by city. If you don't have a physician close to you, find one you can travel to see. It will change your health for the better.

Conclusion

Our bodies are complex electrical machines that are easily damaged by illness, injury, improper diet, lack of sleep, environmental factors, stress, aging, and just the plain wear and tear of living. Choosing the right healthcare treatments when you are experiencing some adversity is a very important decision. I hope you now know you have some options when it comes to choosing the right treatments for your problems. You have a voice and can demand the best possible treatments to cure your diseases. John F Kennedy is quoted as saying, "Change is the law of life. Those who only look to the past and present are certain to miss the future." Don't miss your future by neglecting your healthcare. So much more work needs to be done before Chinese medicine and its modalities are considered mainstream, this can only happen if patients who receive treatments share their experiences with everyone.

A few things you can do to make a difference:

- Write letters to your local and federal government officials, and insurance companies about your concerns about allopathic medicine and benefits from complementary medicine

- Post on social media these same concerns and benefits

- Share your healthcare choices with your friends and family and doctors

- Become a part of the education about changes in healthcare by becoming a healthcare advocate and teaching classes and sharing information any way you can

- Go to Washington, DC and tell your congress and senate representatives what changes in healthcare law you want to see

NOTES

About Me

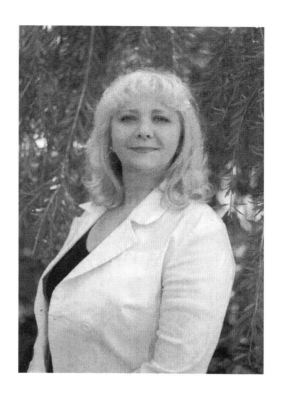

Dr. Brown is an Attorney and an Acupuncture Physician licensed to practice law (Indiana only) and Oriental Medicine and Acupuncture in both Indiana and Florida. She graduated from SUNY Binghamton, Binghamton, NY (1988), Thomas Cooley Law School, Lansing Michigan, (1992) and the Atlantic Institute for Oriental Medicine, Ft Lauderdale, FL (2011). She studied acupuncture and Oriental medicine in Suzhou China for 1.5 years (2006-2008) and NADA protocol at Brighton Hospital, Michigan, (2008) and is a certified Acupuncture Detox Specialist. Dr. Brown has a medical Clinic in Bonita Springs, Florida where she practices acupuncture, injection therapy, homeopathic and herbal medicine, and essential oil application for wellness. She is board certified in acupuncture (NCCAOM) and is a certified DOT medical examiner. As an acupuncture patient and essential oil user, Dr. Brown has seen first-hand the benefits of alternative health care in treating illnesses and improving health and well-being. While living in China with her husband, she was able to explore her interest in acupuncture and Oriental medicine by studying and training with China's best-qualified physicians and acupuncturists. After returning home, Dr. Brown continued her education in acupuncture and has become proficient in the use of essential oils. Dr. Brown has written articles and teaches classes on complementary health care choices and using essential oils for wellness. After suffering from allergies and asthma for years she moved to China and cured herself with Chinese medicine. After returning to the United States she went to medical school at ATOM in Fort Lauderdale, Florida and now practices in Bonita Springs, Florida where she lives with her husband and two dachshunds.

Further Reading

Mini Guide to Acupuncture and Essential Oils, by Dr. Michelle Brown

Acknowledgments

After learning that my brother died from lung cancer at age 53 alone and afraid to tell his family he was sick, it really changed the way I view life and my mission to educate people about complementary medicine. Life is so short, and I knew I had to get started immediately. When I was growing up, I never felt like I was good at anything but after I went to law school, I realized it was my ability to speak for others that I was good at. Law combined with my medical education and experience with western medicine and illness and now my own aging is my driving force to motivate people to start asking questions of doctors about prescriptions and treatment options and start implementing complementary medicine in their healthcare regime.

Thank you so much for reading my book. I hope I will inspire you to make the healthcare changes you need to make today.

Contact me directly or Register for my mailing list at www.anhcare.com

Made in the USA
Columbia, SC
14 October 2021

46846495R10067